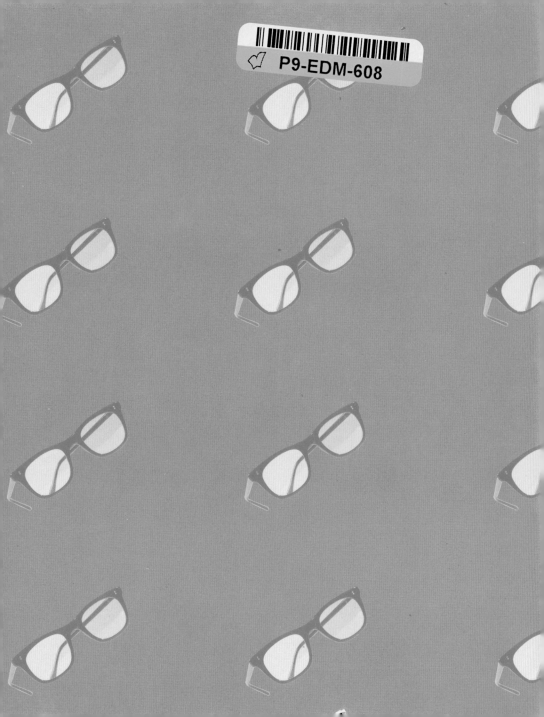

Glasses

Glasses

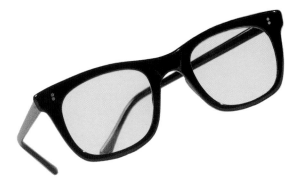

STEWART, TABORI & CHANG

NEW YORK

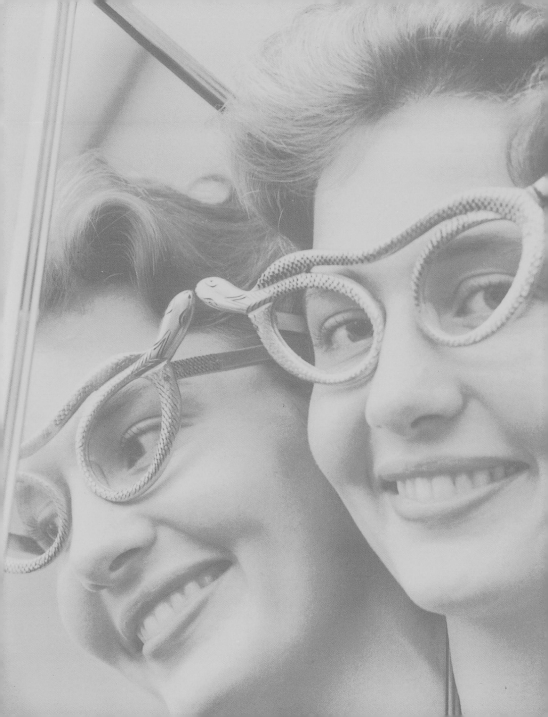

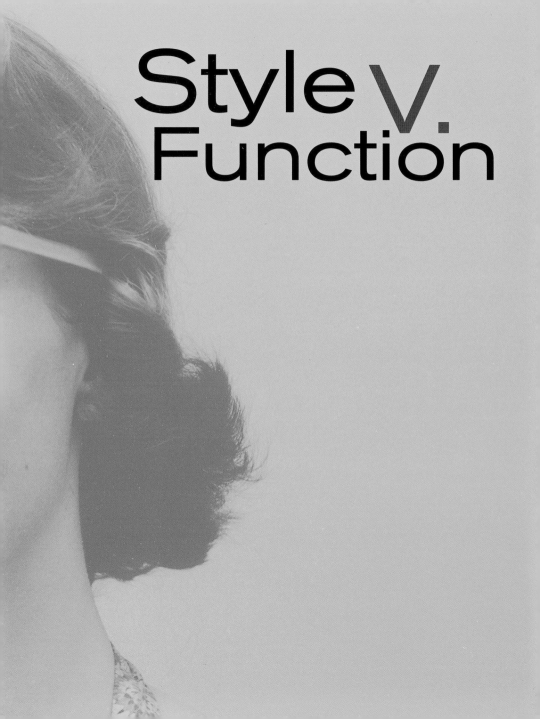

Style V. Function

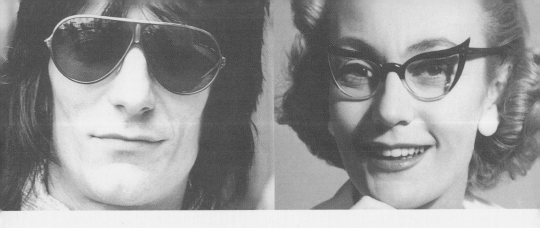

EXUBERANCE

is better than

TASTE.

Gustave Flaubert

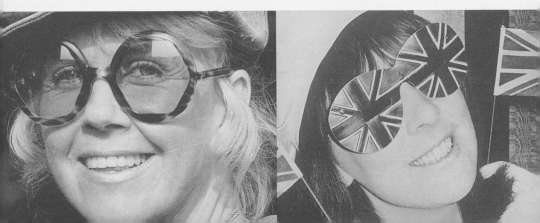

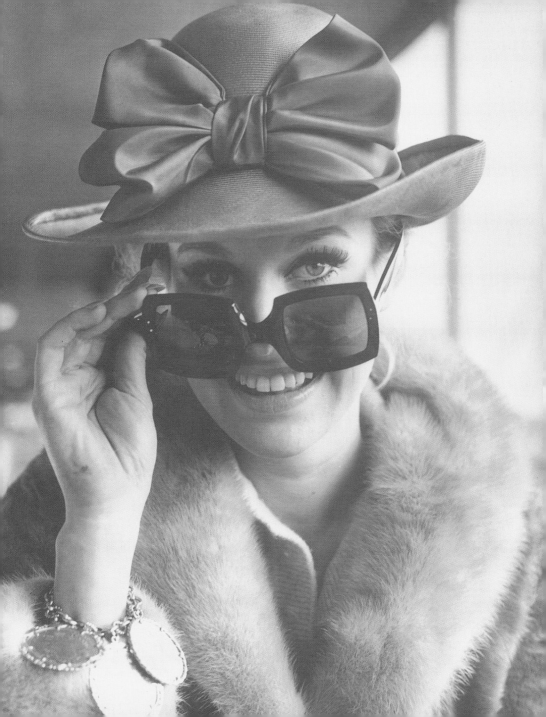

Men seldom make passes at girls who wear glasses.

Dorothy Parker

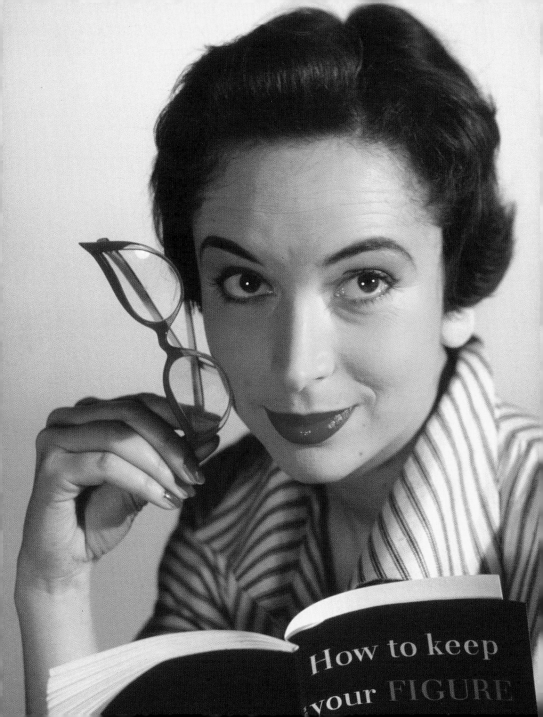

How to keep
your FIGURE

Why Grandma,
what big eyes
you have!

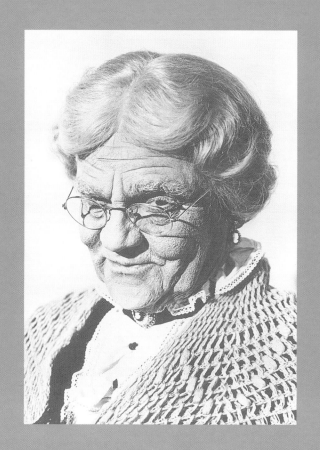

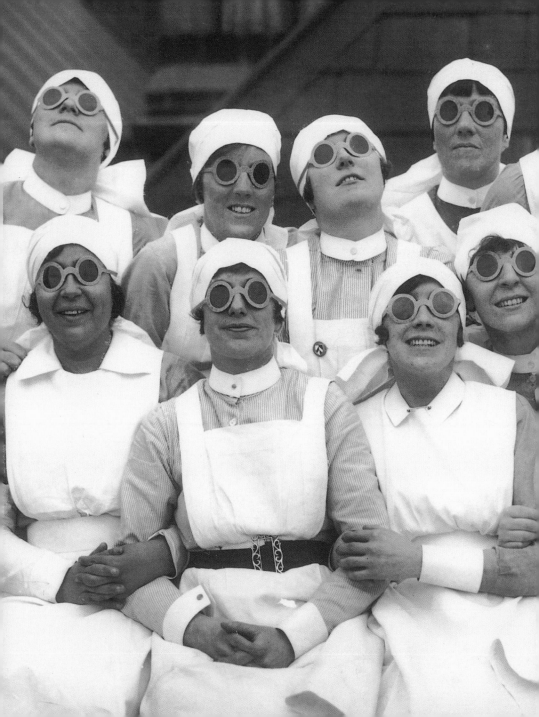

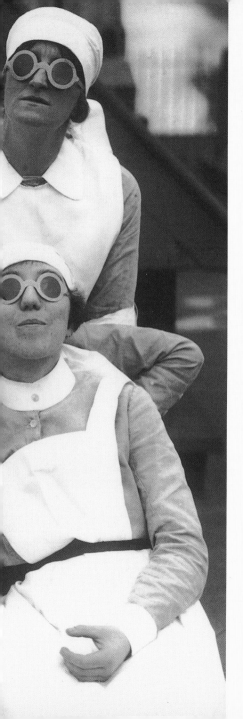

It does not seem
fair that unbeknown
to you every single
item you put on
your body literally
shouts out your
subconscious dreams
and desires to the
whole world.

CYNTHIA HEIMEL

13

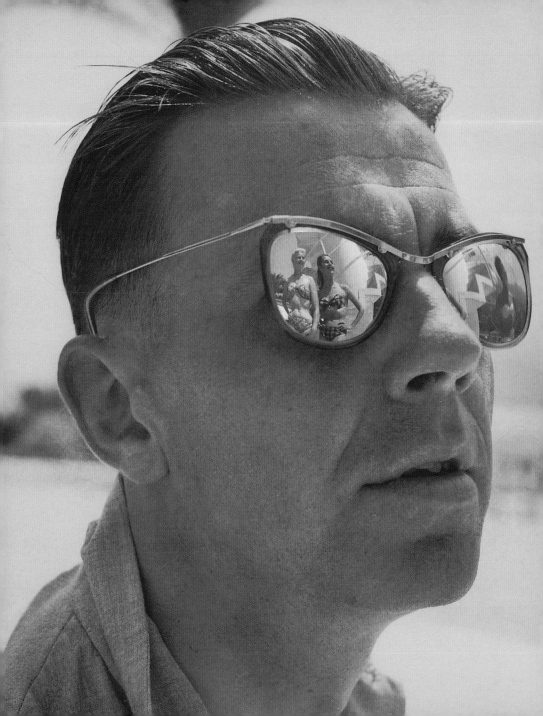

Sun, sea, sand & sex

I have such
poor vision
I can date
anybody.

Garry Shandling

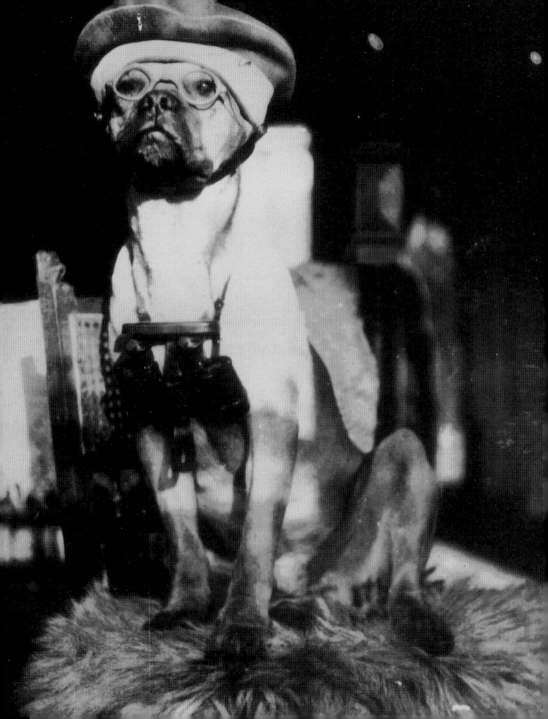

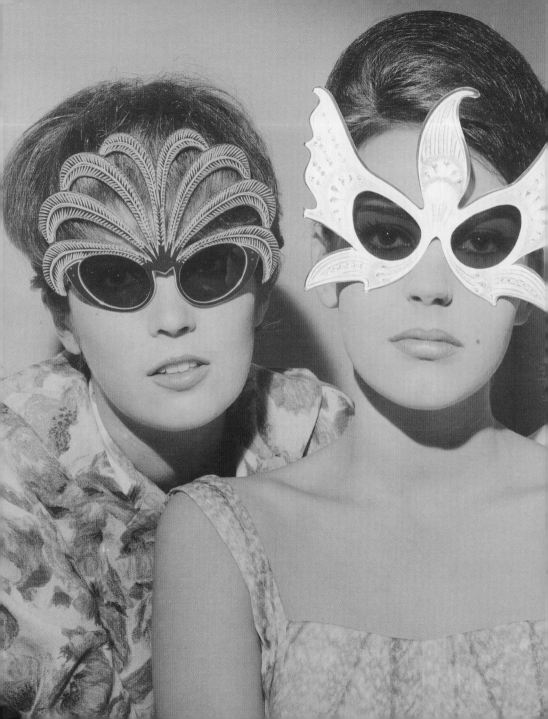

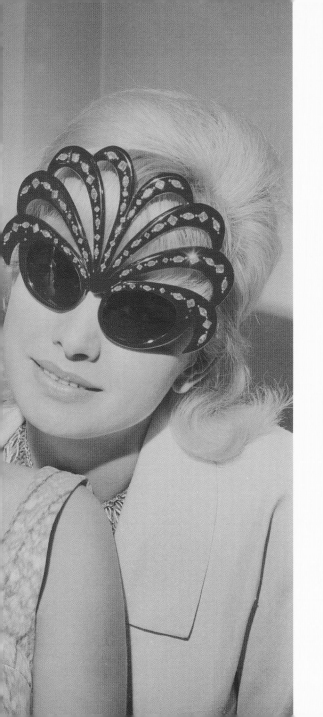

A taste for the grandiose, like a taste for morphia, is, once it has been fully acquired, difficult to keep within limits.

OSBERT LANCASTER

19

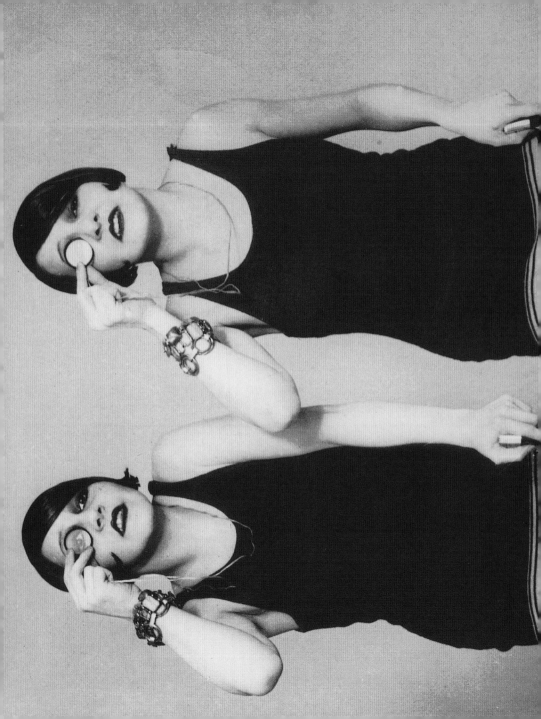

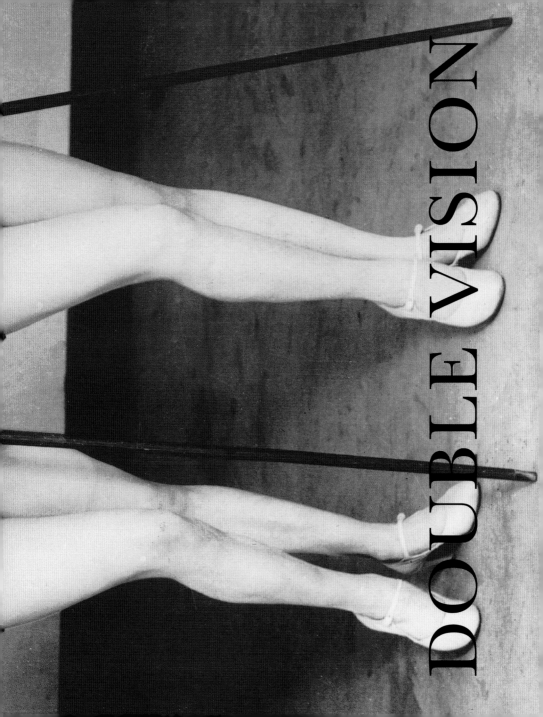

DOUBLE VISION

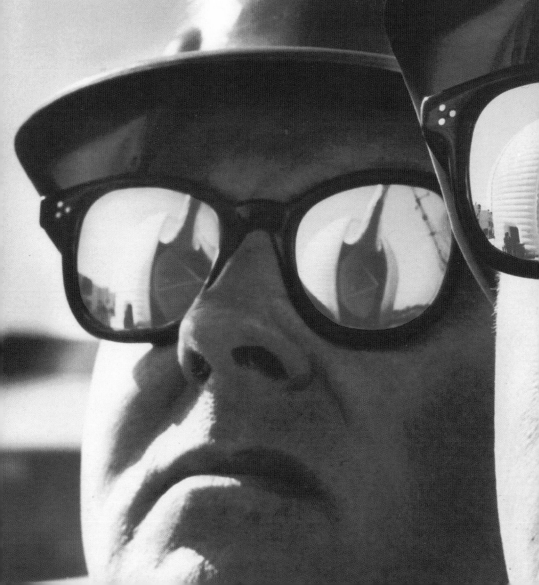

WORK/STRE

NGTH/FORM

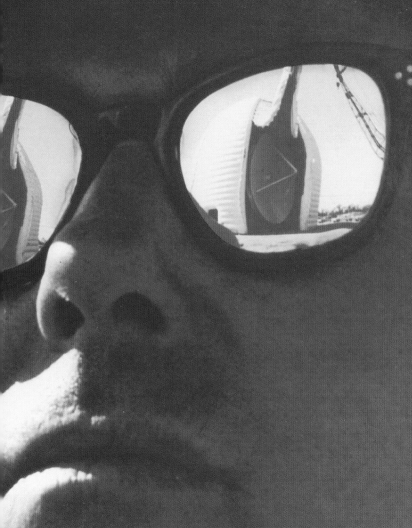

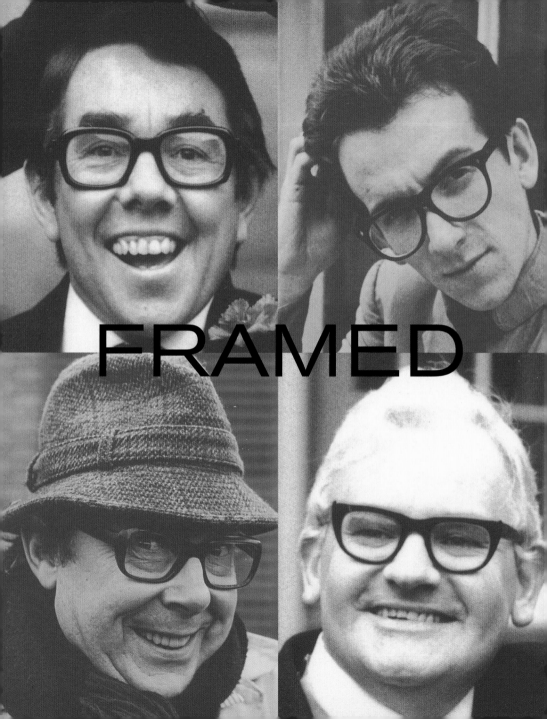

FRAMED

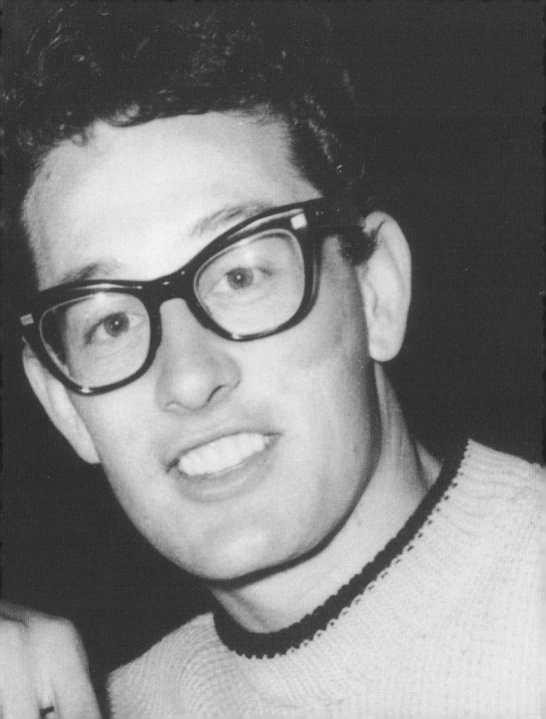

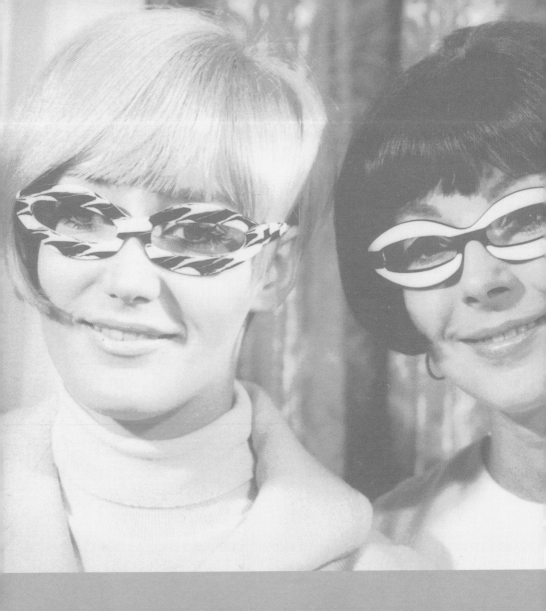

OPTICAL

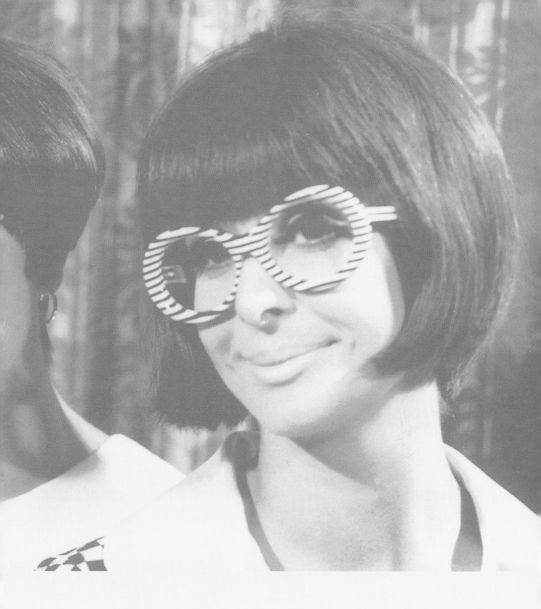

ILLUSION

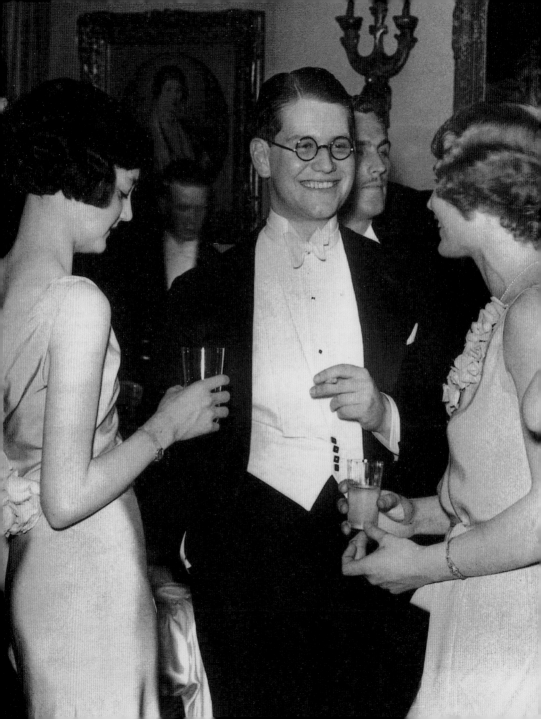

A man who wore a tie that went
twice round the neck was sure,
sooner or later, to inflict some
hideous insult on helpless
womanhood. Add tortoise shell-
rimmed glasses and you had
what practically amounted
to a fiend in human shape.

P.G. Wodehouse, *Mulliner Nights*

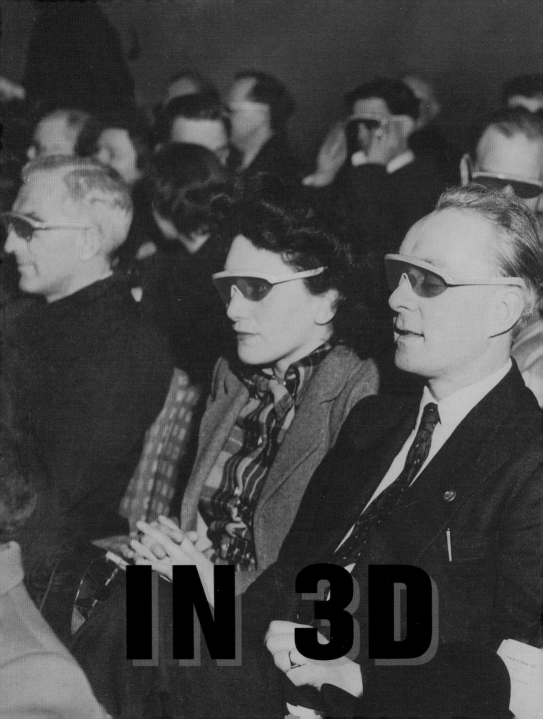

IN 3D

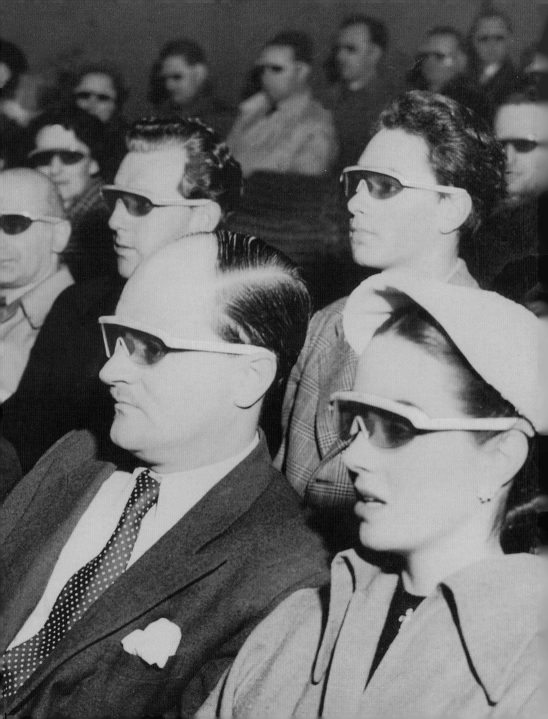

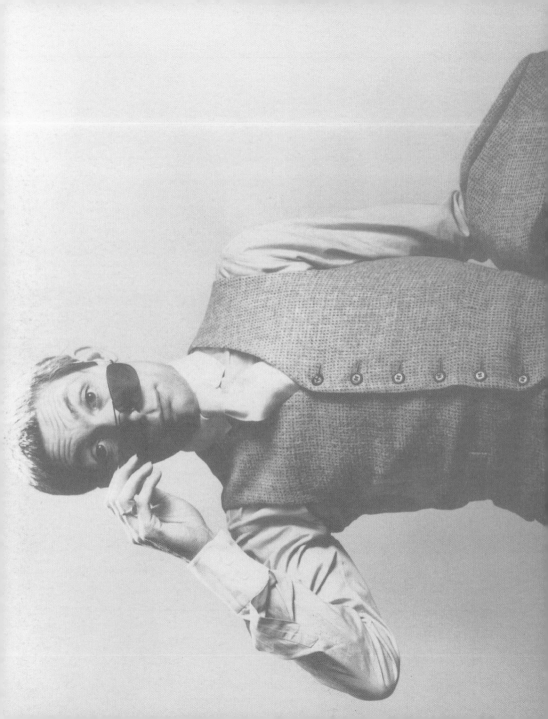

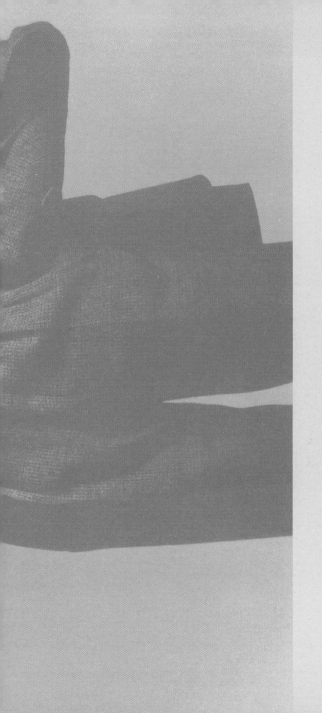

I never wore sunglasses until a few years ago.
I felt I had enough attitude as it was.

FRAN LEBOWITZ

33

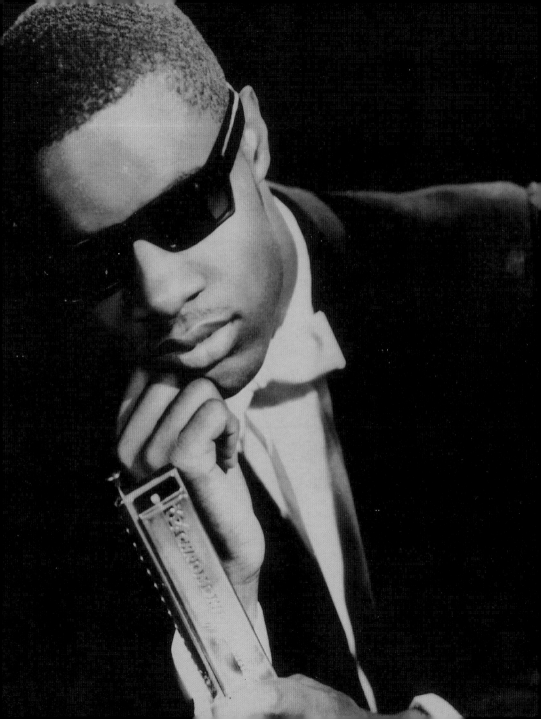

COOL CHARACTERS

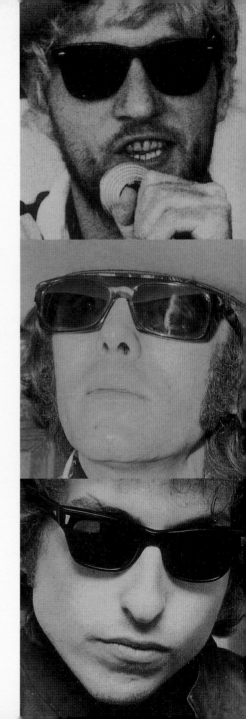

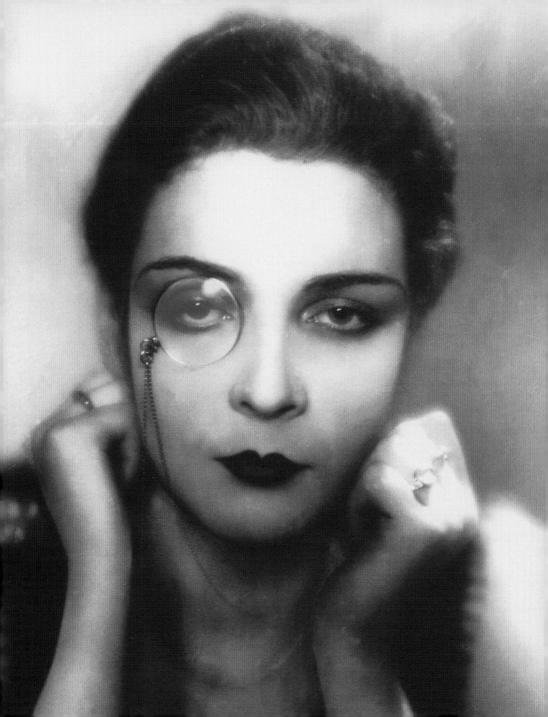

Your Eyes Match Garbo's, Baby, I Wish They Matched Each Other.

Henry Morgan, Song title

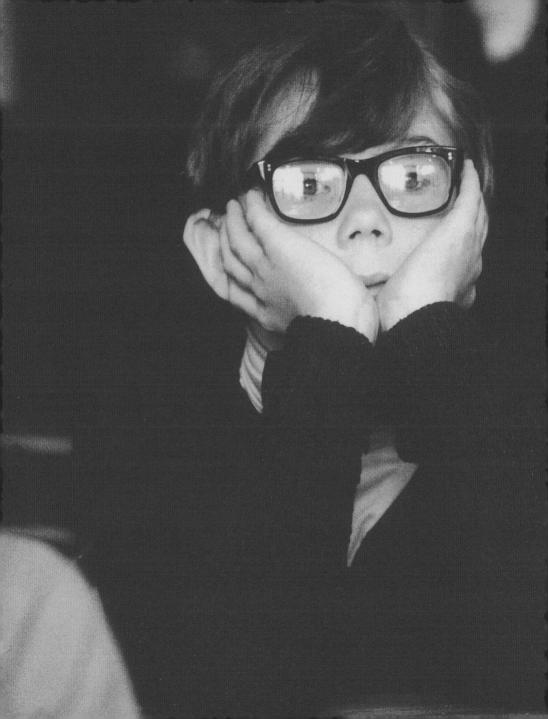

GLAZED OVER

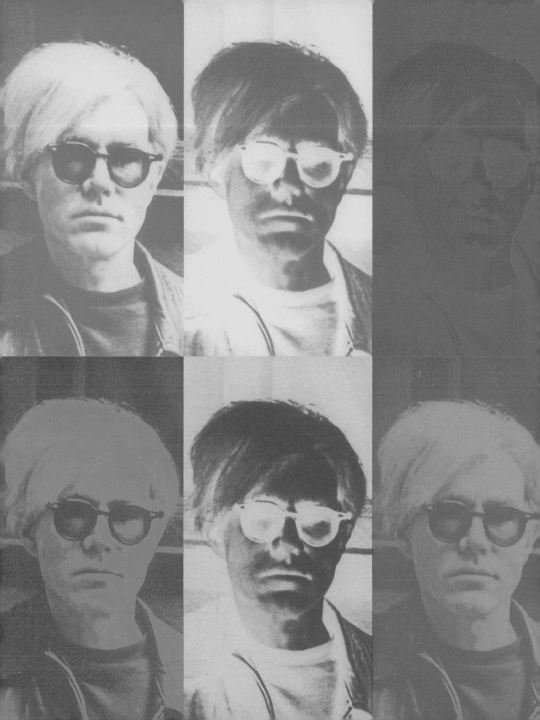

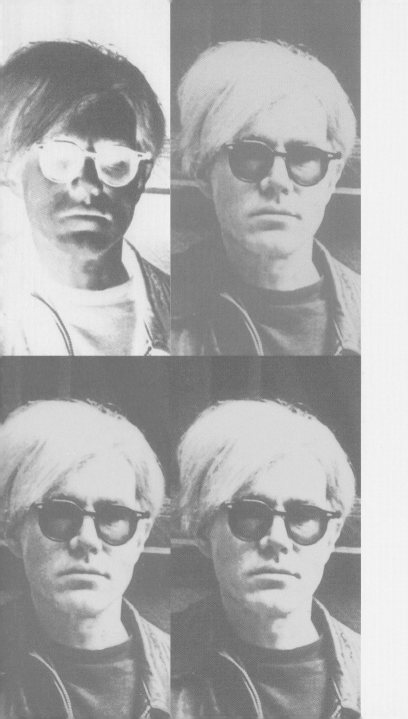

ICON

Save your breath, you may want it to clean your glasses later.

Jules Tannen

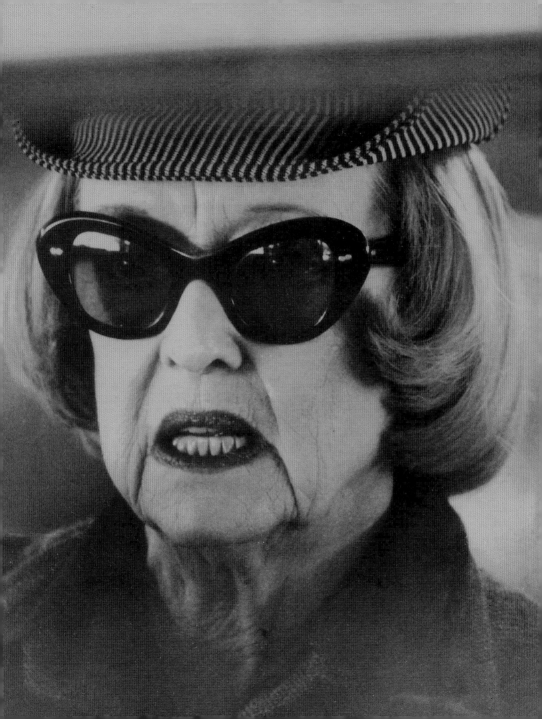

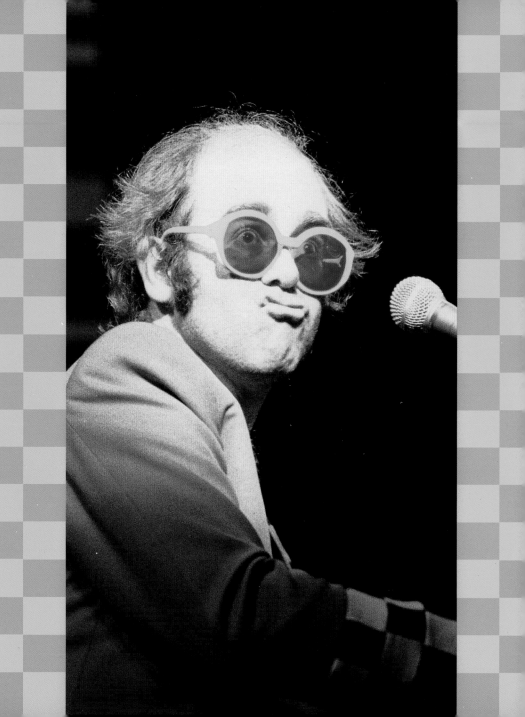

If we wish to succeed, we must make ourselves preposterous.

Crébillon Fils

I never forget a face, but in your case I'll be glad to make an exception.

Groucho Marx

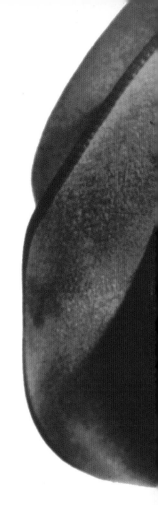

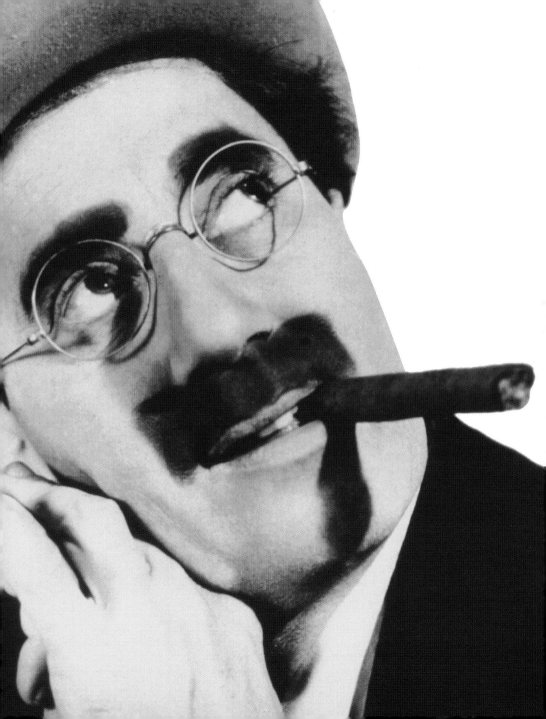

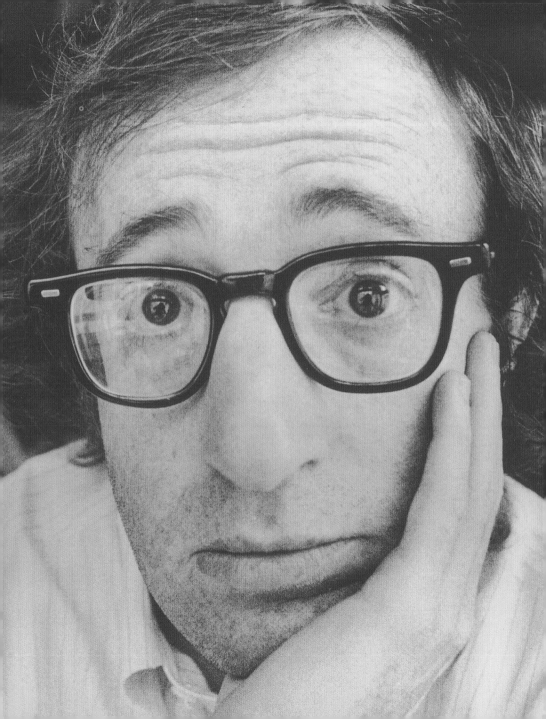

Never hit a man with glasses.

Hit him with your fist.

Anon

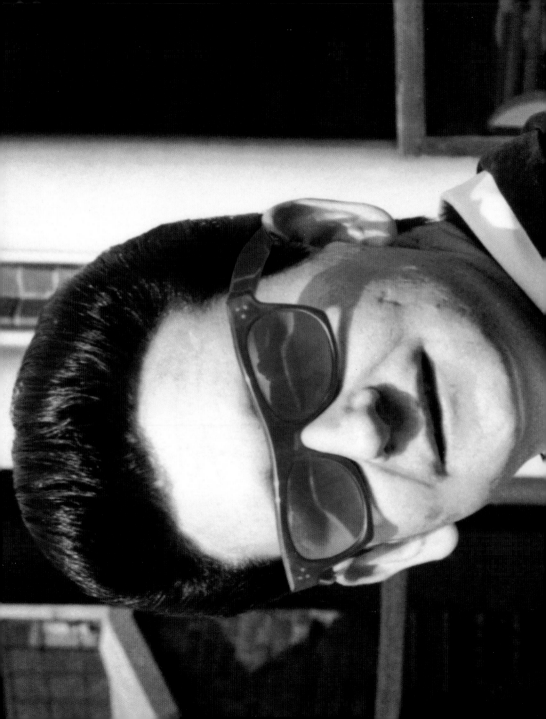

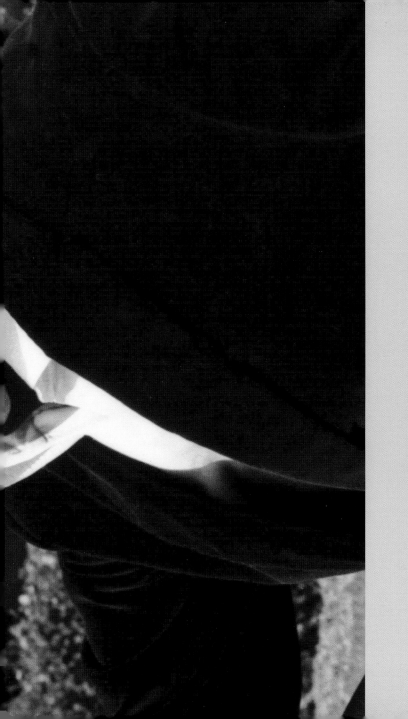

THE BIG O

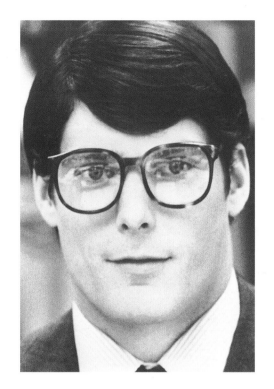

X-RAY
VISION

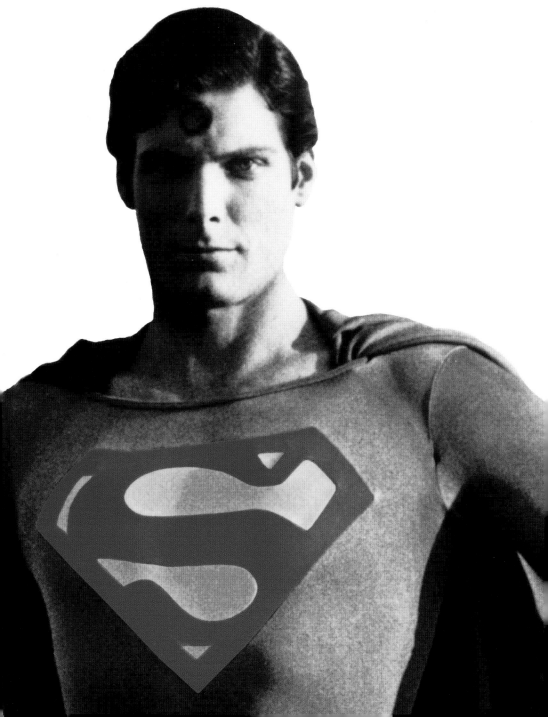

She was never
without dark glasses,
she was always
well groomed, there
was a consequential good
taste in the plainness
of her clothes....

TRUMAN CAPOTE,
BREAKFAST AT TIFFANY'S

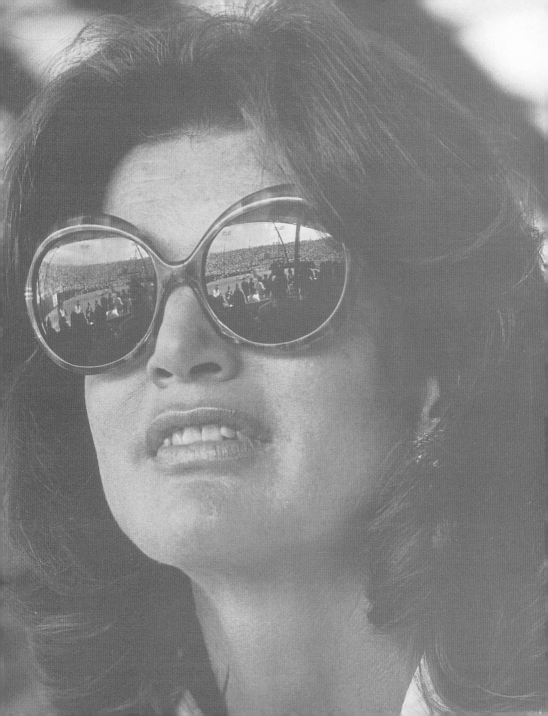

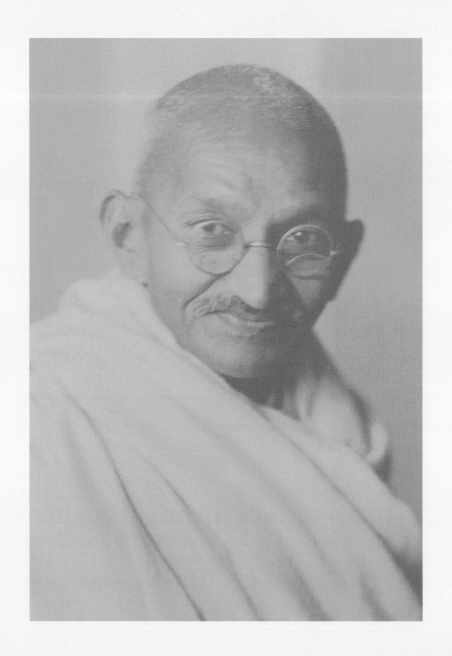

One eye sees,
the other feels.

Paul Klee

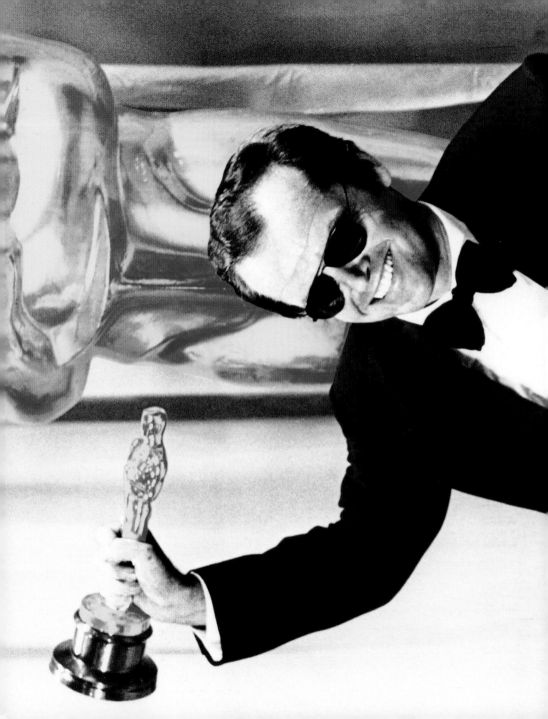

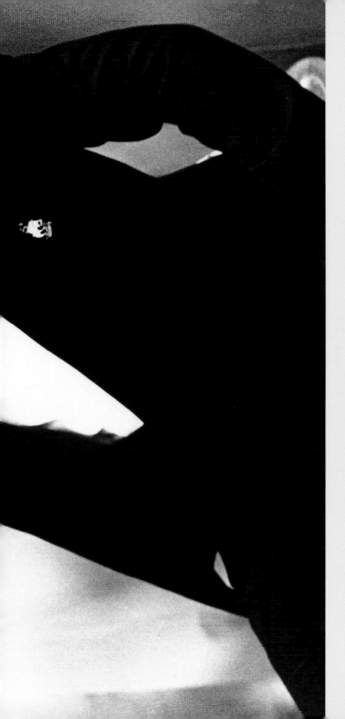

A celebrity is a person who works hard all his life to become well known, then wears dark glasses to avoid being recognized.

Fred Allen

59

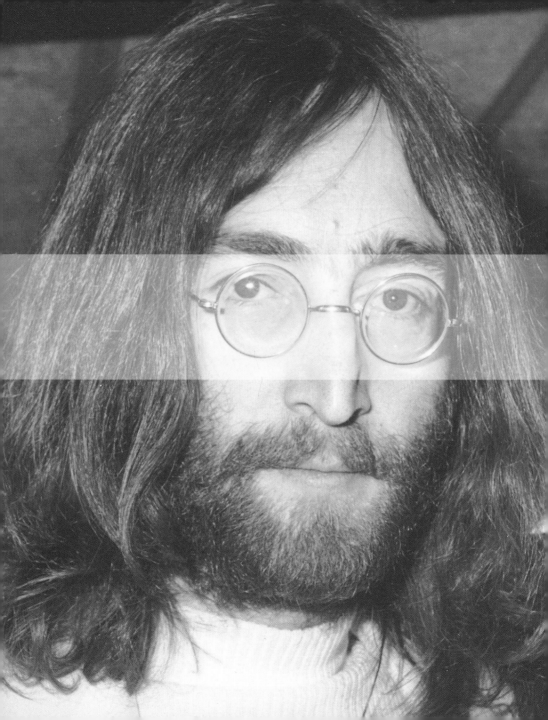

You can't depend on
your eyes when your
imagination is out
of focus.

Mark Twain

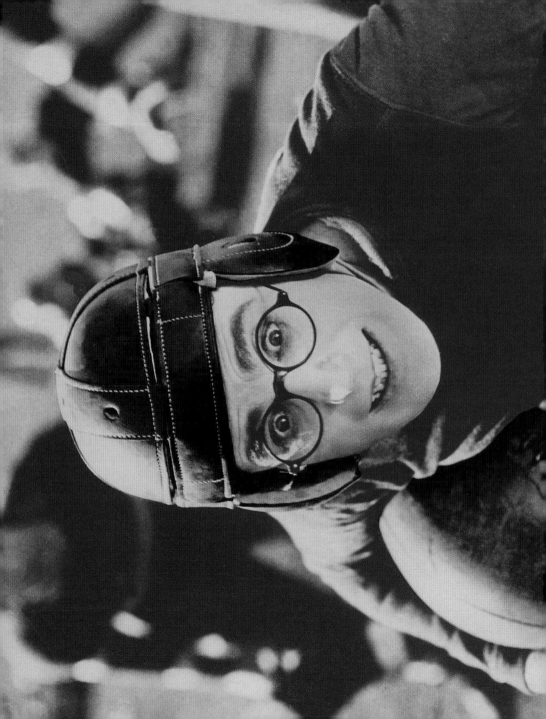

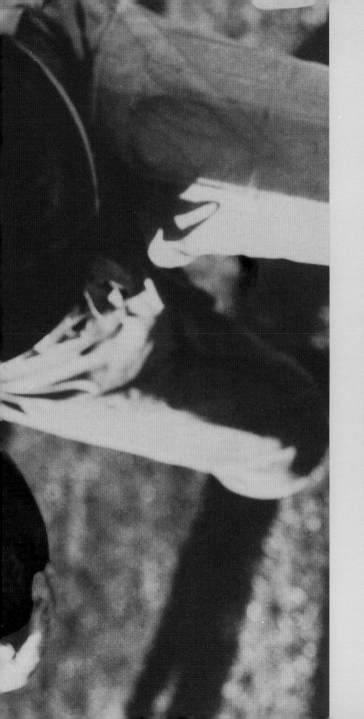

ACTIVE!

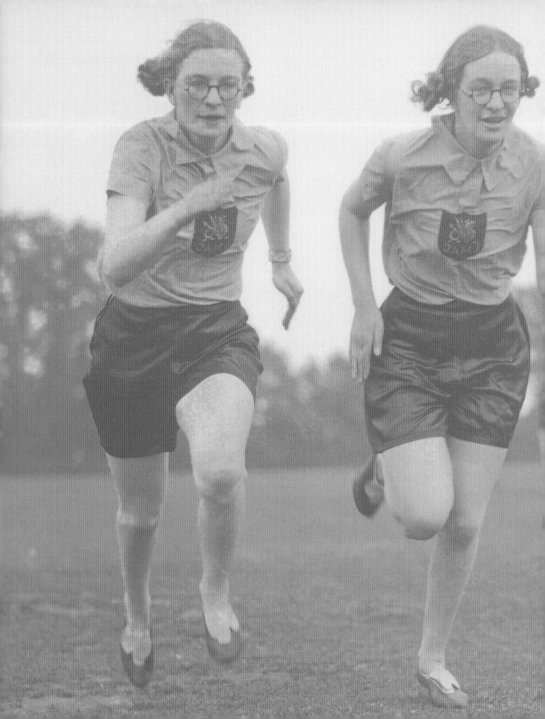

FOUR
EYES

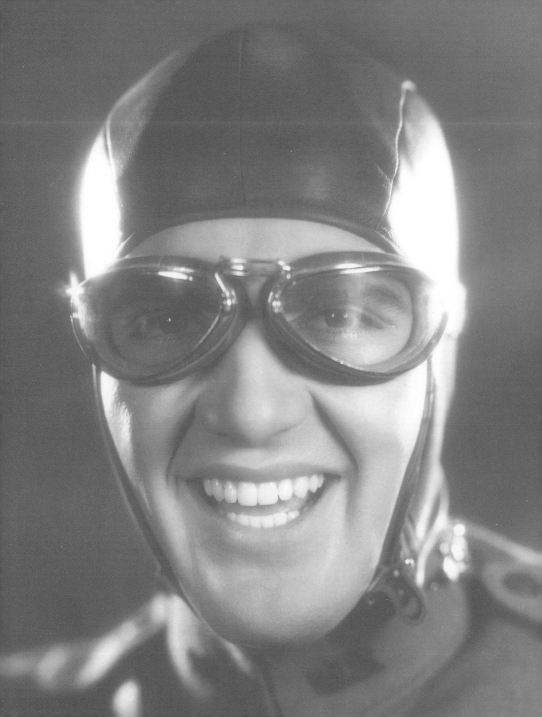

Come fly

with me...

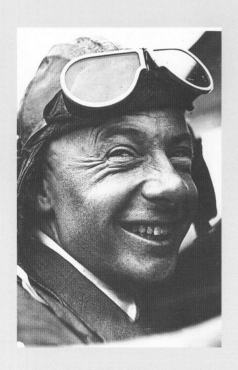

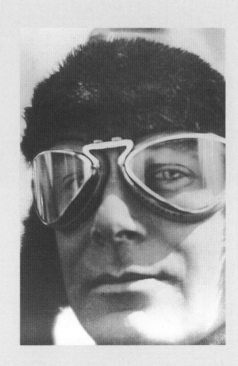

S H A

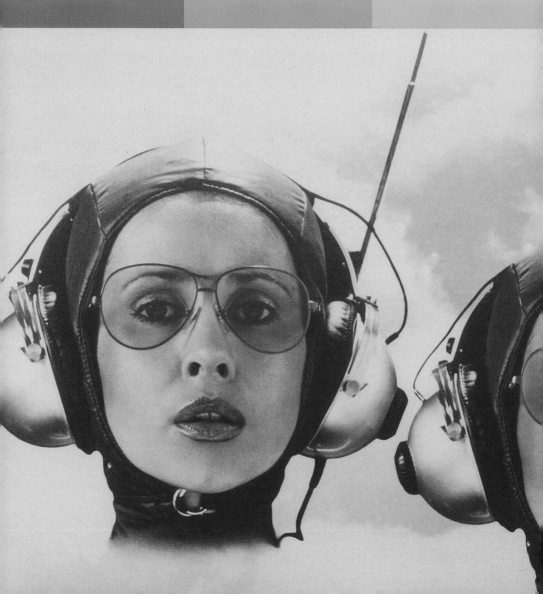

DES

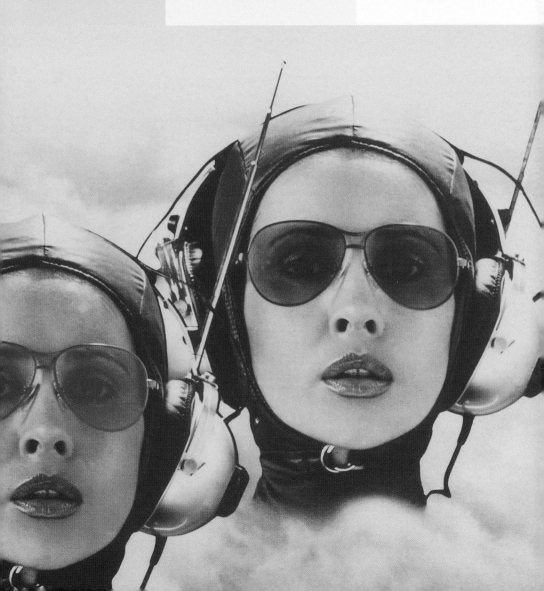

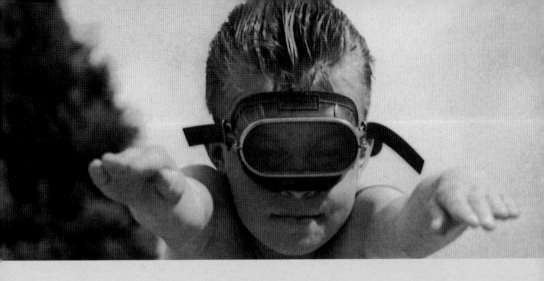

PROTECTIVE
EYE WEAR

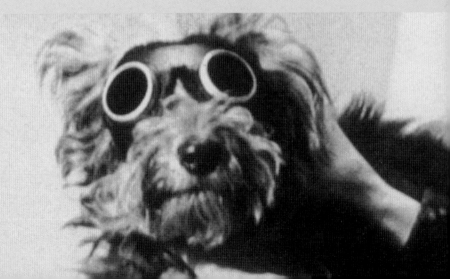

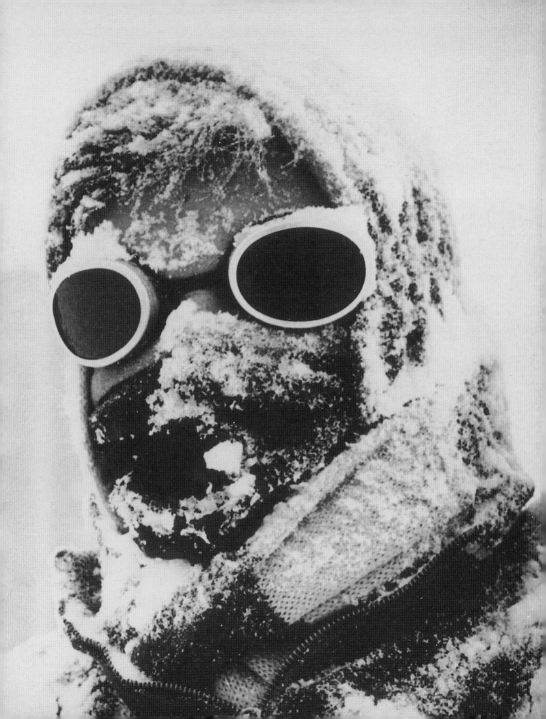

"It's a hundred and six miles to Chicago, we've got a full tank of gas, half a pack of cigarettes, it's dark, and we're wearing sunglasses"
"Hit it"

The Blues Brothers

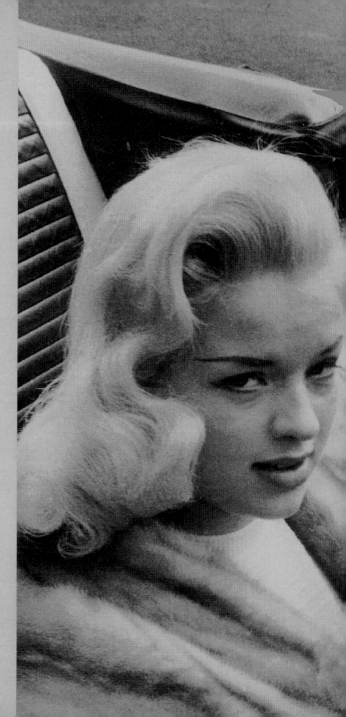

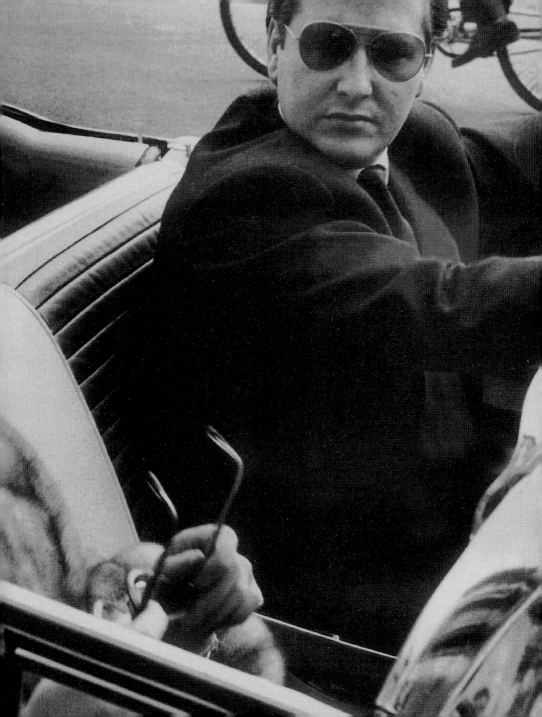

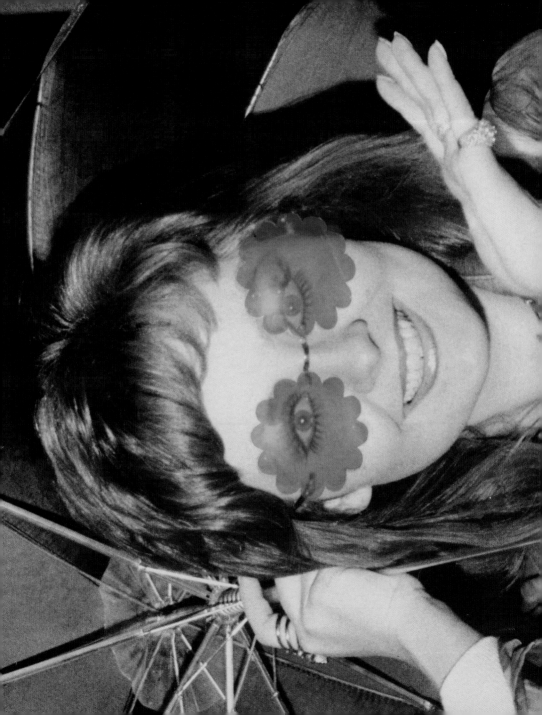

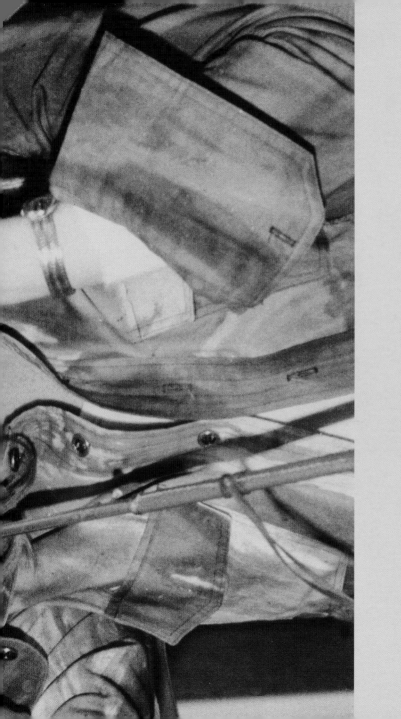

ROSE-TINTED

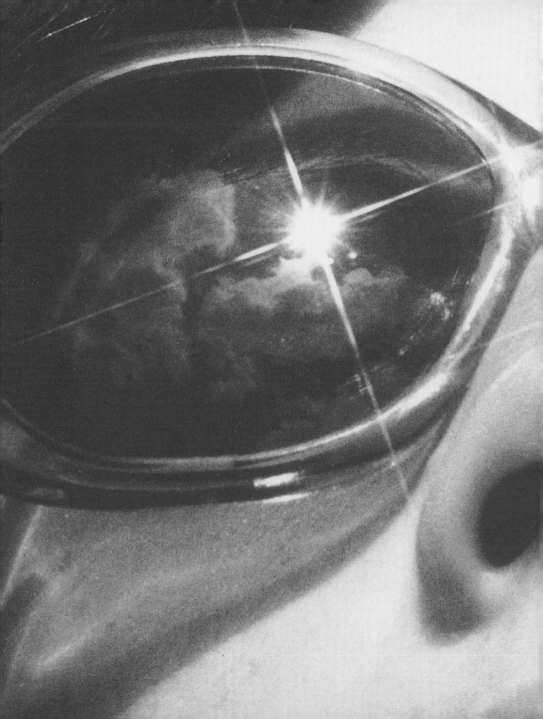

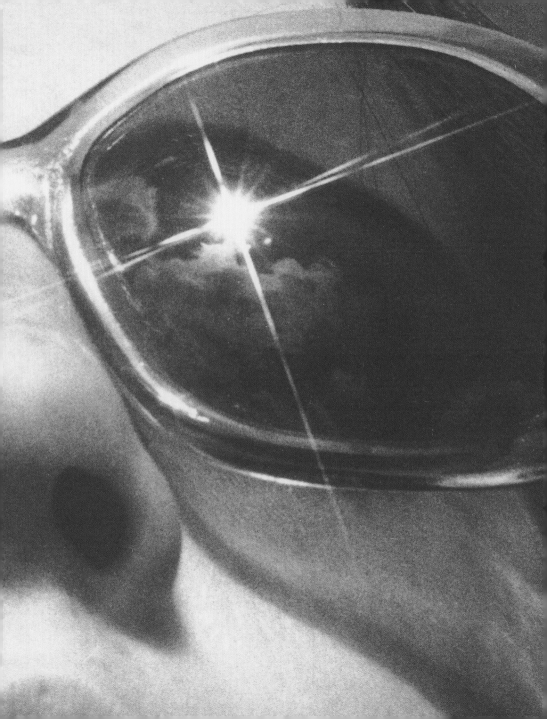

PICTURE CREDITS

All images, except cover and title page, Hulton Getty Picture Collection.

page 4/5: Snake glasses, circa 1956.

page 6: Clockwise from top right, Jean Dawnay, 1956; Samantha Jones, 1966; Doris Day, 1973; Ronnie Wood, 1976.

page 7: Suzanna Leigh, 1965.

page 9: Woman reading a beauty book, 1955.

page 11: James Cagney, 1957.

page 12/13: Nurses observing a solar eclipse through special dark glasses, 1927.

page 14: Man on an Australian beach, 1955.

page 17: German Army dog, circa 1916.

page 18/19: Parisian manequins modelling sunglasses, 1961.

page 20/21: The Dodge Twins, circa 1927.

page 22/23: Engineers, Fullerton, California, 1968.

page 24: Clockwise from top right, Elvis Costello, 1977; Ronnie Barker, 1970; Eric Morcambe, 1979; Ronnie Corbett, 1970.

page 25: Buddy Holly, circa 1957.

page 26/27: Models wearing optical art spectacles, London, 1966.

page 28: Guests chatting over cocktails at the Noble Arts Ball, 1930.

page 30/31: Cinema-goers wearing 3D glasses to view a three dimensional film screened at the Festival of Britain, 1951.

page 32/33: Charlie Watts, drummer with the Rolling Stones, 1983.

page 34: Stevie Wonder, 1979.

page 35: From top to bottom, Captain Sensible, circa 1980; Spencer Dryden, 1968; Bob Dylan, 1966.

page 36: Eva Eras, circa 1930.

page 38/39: Pupil in a classroom at Enfield School, London, 1978.

page 40/41: Andy Warhol, 1967.

page 43: Bette Davis, 1956.

page 44: Elton John, 1977.

46/47: Groucho Marx, circa 1935.

page 48: Woody Allen, 1971.

page 50/51: Roy Orbison, 1964.

page 52: Christopher Reeve as the alter ego of Superman, Clark Kent, 1978.

page 53: Christopher Reeve as Superman, 1978.

page 55: Jackie Onassis, circa 1970.

page 56: Mahatma Gandhi, 1941.

page 58/59: Jack Nicholson with the Oscar that he won for his performance in the film "One Flew Over The Cuckoo's Nest", 1976.

page 60: John Lennon, 1969.

page 62/63: Harold Lloyd, 1925.

page 64/65: Twin sisters G. Eldridge and J. Eldridge competing in the 100 yards, Harrow, Middlesex, 1938.

page 66: Charles Buddy Rogers in the film "Young Eagles", circa 1930.

page 67: From left to right, Charles A. Butler, 1931; Ernst Udet, 1931.

page 68/69: Colormatic light-sensitive sunglasses modelled by the Sunny Girl, 1965.

page 70: From top to bottom, Robert Coles (aged 12) poised to dive, 1953; Dog wearing goggles to protect him from the ultra violet rays used to treat his leg injury, 1949.

page 71: A snow-covered skier, 1938.

page 72/73: Diana Dors with her husband at the Cannes Film Festival, 1956.

page 74/75: British singer Lulu, 1971.

page 76/77: Reflection in sunglasses, 1977.

Published in 1999 by
Stewart, Tabori & Chang
A division of U.S. Media Holdings, Inc.
115 West 18th Street
New York, NY 10011

Distributed in Canada by
General Publishing Company Ltd.
30 Lesmill Road
Don Mills, Ontario, Canada M3B 2T6

Library of Congress Catalog Card Number: 98-88625

ISBN: 1-55670-933-1

Design: John Casey
Series Editor: Elizabeth Carr
Printed in Italy

10 9 8 7 6 5 4 3 2 1

The publishers are grateful to the following authors, agents and publishers for permission to reprint
the following copyright material:

Extract from *Mulliner Nights* by P.G. Wodehouse reprinted by permission of A.P. Watt Ltd. on behalf
of The Trustees of the Wodehouse Estate and Hutchinson as publisher.
Extract from *The Blues Brothers*, copyright © 1999 by Universal City Studios, Inc. Courtesy of
Universal Publishing Rights, a Division of Universal Studios, Inc. All rights reserved.

Every effort has been made to contact copyright holders of material used.
In the case of any accidental infringement, concerned parties are
asked to contact the publishers.

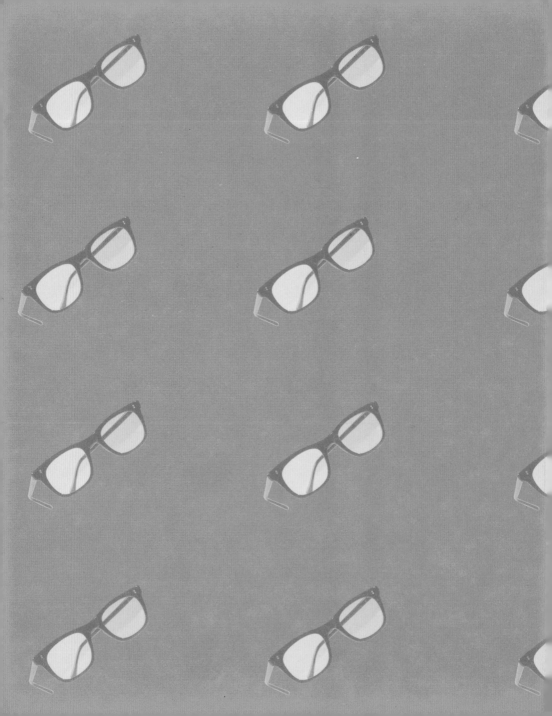